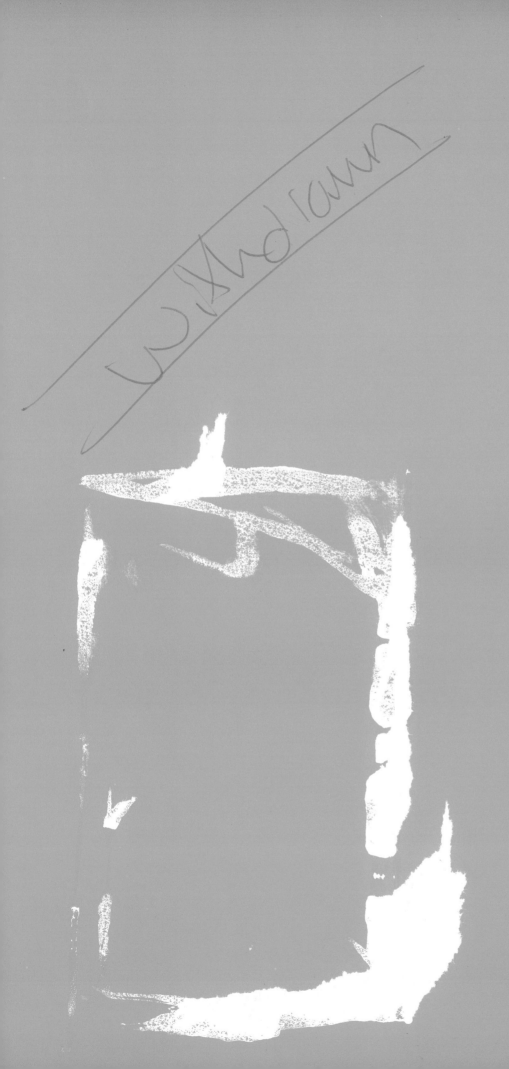

Deafness

© Aladdin Books 1989

Designed and produced by
Aladdin Books Ltd
70 Old Compton Street
London W1V 5PA

First published in
Great Britain in 1989 by
Franklin Watts Ltd
96 Leonard Street
London EC2A 4RH

Design: David West Children's Book Design
Editor: Zuza Vrbova
Picture Research: Cecilia Weston-Baker
Illustrator: Stuart Brendon

Consultant: Colin Redman on behalf of The National Deaf
Children's Society

ISBN 0-7496-0042-X

Printed in Belgium

CONTENTS

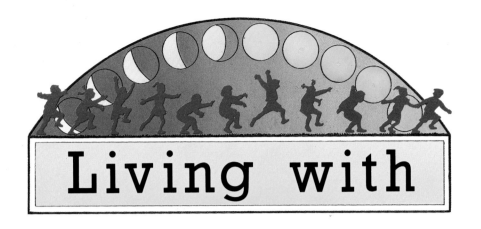

Living with

Deafness

Barbara Taylor

FRANKLIN WATTS
London : New York : Toronto : Sydney

HOW THE EAR WORKS

The ear collects vibrations from the air (sounds) and changes them into nerve impulses, which the brain "hears." The outer ear is made up of the pinna and the ear canal. Near its entrance, the ear canal is lined with hairs and wax, which help to keep it clean.

The ear canal leads to a flexible, circular membrane, called the eardrum. When sound waves hit the eardrum, it vibrates. This makes three tiny bones in the middle ear vibrate. These bones make the vibrations stronger and more intensified and pass them on to the inner ear.

The inner ear consists of a complex system of tubes filled with a watery liquid. Vibrations from the middle ear make the liquid move, and sensitive nerve endings convert this movement into electrical signals. These signals are sent to the brain along the nerve of hearing (auditory nerve).

The way in which the electrical signals are interpreted by the brain is not yet clearly understood.

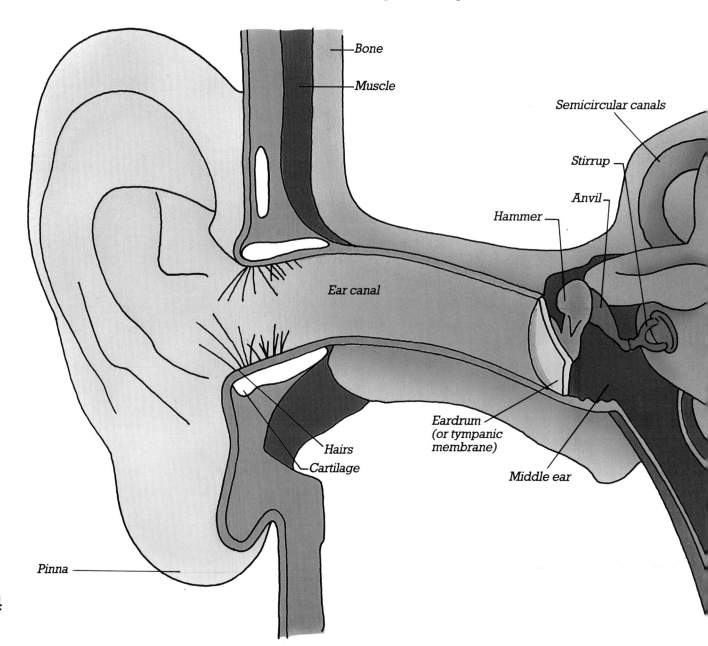

Bone

Muscle

Semicircular canals

Stirrup

Anvil

Hammer

Ear canal

Eardrum (or tympanic membrane)

Hairs

Cartilage

Middle ear

Pinna

Seeing sound

Sounds are made when something makes the air shake backwards and forwards very fast. These shaking movements are called vibrations. When air molecules vibrate, they bump against each other. This causes the vibrations to spread through the air in waves – called sound.

Sound waves are invisible but you can see evidence of them if you hold a vibrating tuning fork in some water. The sound waves make the water shake and splash (below).

Feeling sound

The sounds we make come from the throat. Put one hand against the front of your throat and make a humming noise. Can you feel your throat vibrating? In the same way you can feel the sound of a drum skin vibrating (below). Inside the throat are folds of muscle called vocal cords. When we want to speak or sing, we push air from the lungs past the vocal cords. This makes the cords vibrate and produce sounds. The sounds are shaped into words by your mouth and tongue.

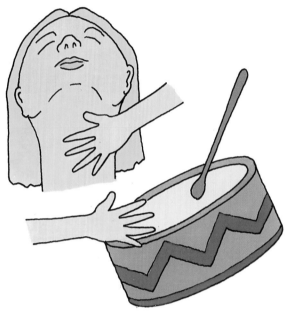

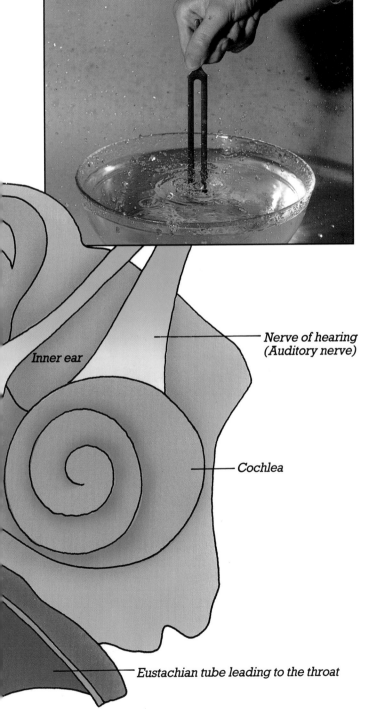

Inner ear

*Nerve of hearing
(Auditory nerve)*

Cochlea

Eustachian tube leading to the throat

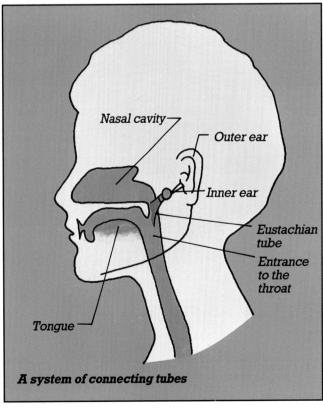

Nasal cavity

Outer ear

Inner ear

Eustachian tube

Entrance to the throat

Tongue

A system of connecting tubes

5

The smallest bones

The three bones in the middle ear are the smallest bones in the body. Because of their shape, they are called the hammer, anvil and stirrup. They are linked so that the vibrations of one bone can easily make the next bone in the chain vibrate and so send signals to the brain.

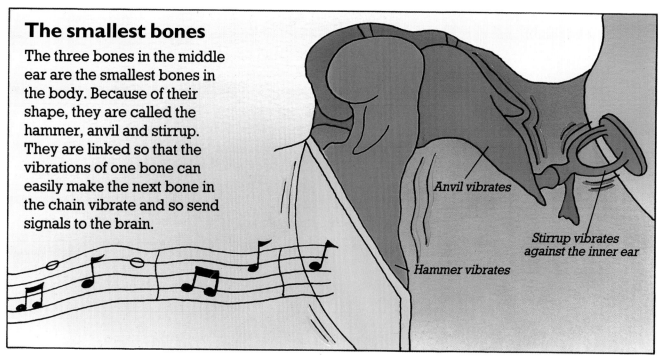

Anvil vibrates

Stirrup vibrates against the inner ear

Hammer vibrates

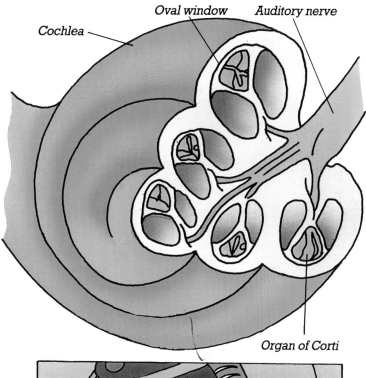

Cochlea

Oval window

Auditory nerve

Organ of Corti

Sound waves into signals

In the spiral cochlea of the inner ear, the vibrations caused by sound waves in the air are converted into electrical signals. Vibrations enter the cochlea through a membrane called the oval window. They pass into a fluid-filled tube. Altogether it is about as long as your little finger and it is shaped like a snail's shell. The tube contains membranes with thousands of tiny, hair-like nerve endings. This is called the organ of Corti. The vibrations make the fluid move, which bends the hairs and causes the nerves to fire off electrical signals. These signals are sent to the brain along the auditory nerve. Bigger vibrations create louder sounds.

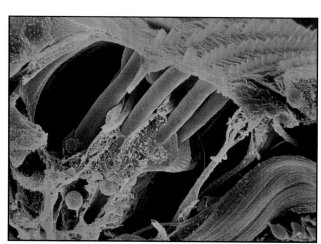

6 *Sensory hair cells in the organ of Corti*

Electron micrograph of the organ of Corti

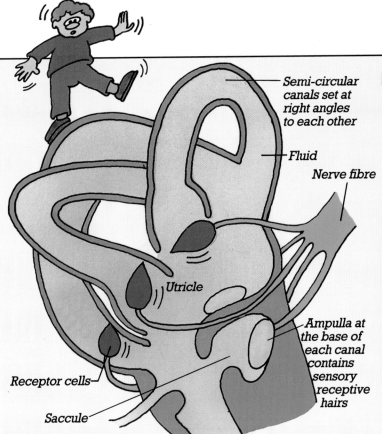

Semi-circular
canals set at
right angles
to each other

Fluid

Nerve fibre

Utricle

Ampulla at
the base of
each canal
contains
sensory
receptive
hairs

Receptor cells

Saccule

BALANCE

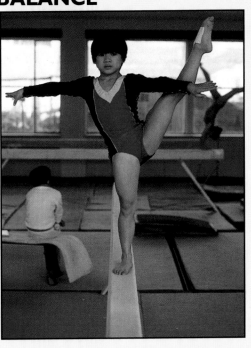

It is the three semi-circular canals, in the inner ear, that give you your sense of balance. At one end of each is a swollen area called the ampulla. The semi-circular canals open into two sacs called the utricle and the saccule. The whole structure is filled with fluid. The ampulla, utricle and saccule all contain sensory hairs. As you tilt your head, the fluid presses on the hairs, which convert the pressure into electrical signals that travel to the brain. The sacs tell you the position of your head and the canals tell you the direction it is moving. In the utricle and saccule, the tiny hairs are surrounded by a jelly-like substance containing minute crystals of calcium carbonate, called otoliths. As the crystals move, under the influence of gravity, they stimulate the hairs, which trigger nerve impulses to the brain.

HEARING AND THE BRAIN

Signals from the cochlea in the inner ear travel to the brain along the auditory nerve. The nerve carries the sound signals to the base of the brain. This area is called the auditory cortex. Here the brain interprets the signals into "sounds". The way in which sound waves picked up by our ears are actually turned into electrical energy, and interpreted by the brain, is not fully understood.

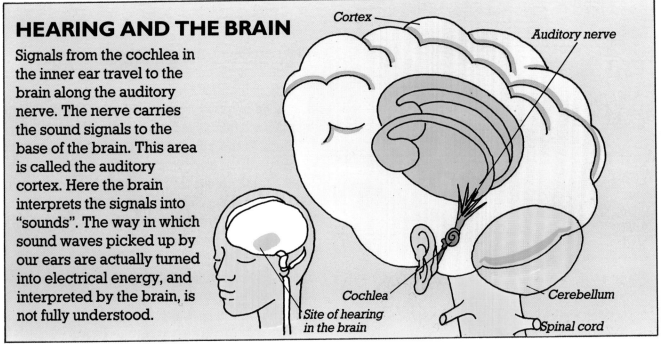

Cortex

Auditory nerve

Cochlea

Cerebellum

Site of hearing
in the brain

Spinal cord

7

KINDS OF HEARING PROBLEMS

At least one child in every thousand is born profoundly deaf. Many more people develop hearing impediments later in life because of accidents or diseases.

There are two main kinds of hearing problem. One kind affects the outer or middle ear. This can produce a "conductive" hearing difficulty and it can usually be treated and cured. The other main type of problem that affects people's sense of hearing is connected to the inner ear or the nerve of hearing (auditory nerve). It is called "nerve deafness". Unfortunately, this kind of deafness is usually permanent.

Conductive deafness leads to a loss of loudness, which is like trying to listen to someone who is speaking very quietly or is very far away. Nerve deafness cuts down the loudness and distorts sounds as well. So it is rather like listening to someone speaking an unknown foreign language. This disordered interpretation of sound is a typical symptom of inner ear diseases.

Blocked ears

One of the simplest causes of hearing loss is the ear canal becoming blocked. This stops some sound waves from reaching the eardrum. Natural wax moves out of the ear all the time to help carry dirt out of the ear. But if this wax becomes hard, it stays in the canal and forms a blockage. A small object which has been pushed into the ear can also block out sound. Because the ear canal is lined with skin, it can also be blocked by skin conditions such as eczema or boils.

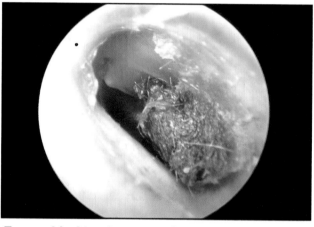

Ear wax blocking the ear canal

Glue ear

Fluid produced in the middle ear usually drains down a tube that leads to the throat. This is called the Eustachian tube. If the Eustachian tube becomes blocked by an infection or enlarged adenoids, infected fluid collects in the middle ear. The fluid may become thick and sticky so this problem is also called "glue ear". The "glue" makes it harder for the eardrum and the bones in the middle ear to vibrate properly.

The Eustachian tube lets air from outside into the middle ear. This keeps the air pressure the same on both sides of the eardrum. A blocked Eustachian tube causes air pressure to build up inside the ear. This pressure may damage the eardrum.

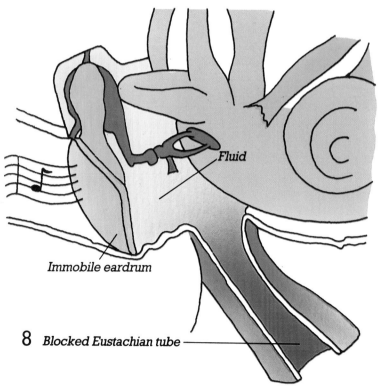

Fluid

Immobile eardrum

Blocked Eustachian tube

Damaged eardrum

If a person has several serious infections in the middle ear, the eardrum becomes weaker. Eventually, holes or perforations may appear in it. The holes stop the eardrum from vibrating normally and lead to a loss of hearing. Holes in the eardrum usually heal naturally, but if the infection is serious and goes on for a long time, the holes may stay open. This may need special repair treatment. (The medical name for this condition is *chronic otitis media*).

Holes in the eardrum may also be caused by poking things into the ear, a serious blow to the ear, or very loud noises, such as explosions.

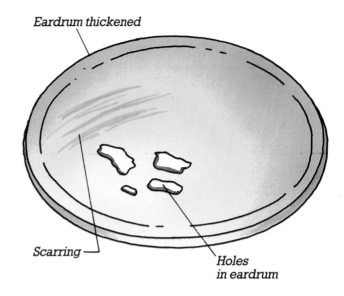

Eardrum thickened

Scarring

Holes
in eardrum

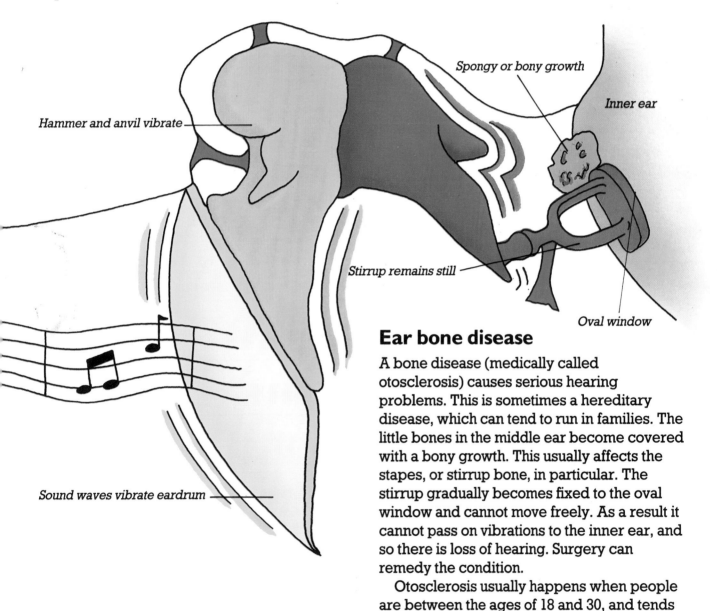

Hammer and anvil vibrate

Spongy or bony growth

Inner ear

Stirrup remains still

Oval window

Sound waves vibrate eardrum

Ear bone disease

A bone disease (medically called otosclerosis) causes serious hearing problems. This is sometimes a hereditary disease, which can tend to run in families. The little bones in the middle ear become covered with a bony growth. This usually affects the stapes, or stirrup bone, in particular. The stirrup gradually becomes fixed to the oval window and cannot move freely. As a result it cannot pass on vibrations to the inner ear, and so there is loss of hearing. Surgery can remedy the condition.

Otosclerosis usually happens when people are between the ages of 18 and 30, and tends to become more serious as people become older. It is more common in women.

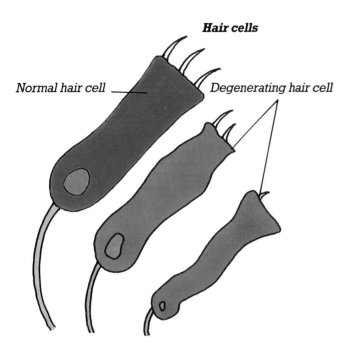

Normal hair cell — *Hair cells* — *Degenerating hair cell*

Nerve deafness

Nerve deafness may develop at any time from before birth through to old age. The cochlea is a very sensitive organ and can be damaged by genetic factors, childhood diseases, very loud noises and some drugs. Most elderly people have some form of nerve deafness.

A difficult or premature birth, particularly when the baby does not receive enough oxygen, can cause nerve deafness. Scientists do not understand how this happens. At birth, a baby may develop jaundice, which can damage the auditory nerve and lead to hearing loss. Jaundice is more likely in premature babies. Many of the problems that may occur during birth are becoming less common as better techniques are developed for caring for "at risk" babies.

Tinnitus

Buzzing or ringing noises in the ears – called tinnitus – affect many people, although the reason for the noises is not clearly understood. It is often hard for a person to work out where in the hearing system the noises are coming from. Some people find the noises almost unbearable. It often occurs in elderly people.

Tinnitus may be caused by very loud noise as well as infections and diseases of the ear. Some people feel that certain drugs and some kinds of food and drink seem to make the noises more unbearable. A person can experience tinnitus without deafness and it can be painful at times.

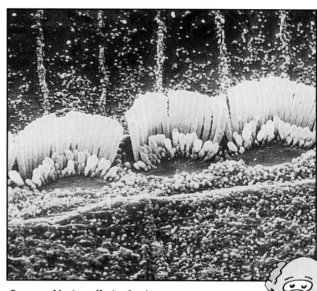

A row of hair cells in the inner ear

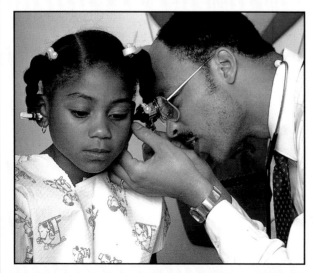

AN EAR EXAMINATION

A doctor can look into the outer ear and the eardrum with an instrument called an auroscope. With an auroscope, a doctor can see if there is a blockage in the ear canal. He or she can also examine the eardrum to see if there are any holes in the surface or if the eardrum is swollen and out of shape. An infection in the middle ear makes the eardrum bulge outwards and look red and sore. A surgeon who specializes in problems of the ear is an otologist.

CHILDHOOD DISEASES

Diseases in childhood may cause severe hearing loss. They include viral diseases such as measles and mumps as well as meningitis, typhoid fever and diphtheria. Any hearing loss tends to occur suddenly at the time of the disease.

Fortunately, only a small number of the people who have these diseases develop a hearing problem. The mumps virus is unusual because it almost always affects one ear only. The other ear remains perfectly normal. The German measles (rubella) virus can affect the developing ears of a baby in the womb.

A problem only occurs if a bacterial infection damages the cochlea or if a viral infection attacks the hearing nerve.

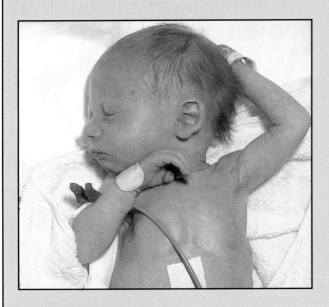

Meningitis

Meningitis causes the membrane covering the brain to become inflamed. If the infection reaches the throat, nose and ears it may destroy the snail-like organ of Corti, in the inner ear, and the auditory nerve.

Measles

Measles may lead to an infection in the middle ear, or the virus may damage the cochlea. This kind of complication can occur as a direct result of the measles infection and a vaccine can prevent such serious consequences.

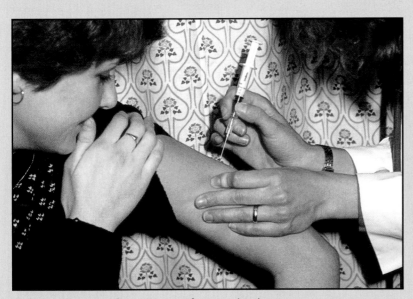

Girl being given a German measles vaccination

Vaccinations

If a woman has German measles (rubella) for the first time during pregnancy, part of the baby's cochlea may be destroyed. So her baby will be born with nerve deafness. The risks are greatest in early pregnancy. Fortunately, there is now a vaccination that gives children protection against rubella, mumps and measles. It is called an MMR vaccination and is given to all children in the UK.

11

TREATMENT FOR EAR PROBLEMS

Hearing loss in the outer or middle ear can be treated with drugs to clear up infections. Operations may sometimes be necessary to repair holes in the eardrum or drain infected fluid out of the middle ear. Bone diseases can be treated by replacing the stapes (or stirrup) bone with an artifical one.

It is impossible to cure nerve deafness in the inner ear. But adults or older people, rather than children, can have a cochlear implant. This is a sophisticated hearing aid in which tiny electrodes are implanted in or on the cochlea. This kind of operation relies on the memory of sound and may improve hearing for some people who have become profoundly deaf.

Hearing aids make sounds louder and help people with a hearing impairment to cope with life at home, at school or at work. Hearing aids are worn on the body or behind the ear (these are sometimes called post-aural aids). Radio aids provide a direct link from one person to another.

Detecting deafness in babies

It is difficult to test the hearing of a newborn baby because babies can only respond in a limited way and the responses vary. But a device called an auditory cradle can measure a baby's breathing pattern in response to sound (top right). This does not measure hearing levels or show where a problem is. But it does indicate possible problems, so the baby can be watched carefully and any hearing impediment can be treated.

All babies should have their hearing tested when they are between six and nine months old (lower right). At this age, they can hold up their heads without help. If they hear a sound which is made behind them, they are able to turn towards the sound. This is called distraction testing. The tester makes the sounds at a low level at first but, if the baby does not turn round, the level is increased until he or she responds.

Ear infections are a very common condition in babies and toddlers who may not even complain of earache but simply feel unwell, with perhaps a temperature. For this reason doctors always examine the ears of young children who have a fever.

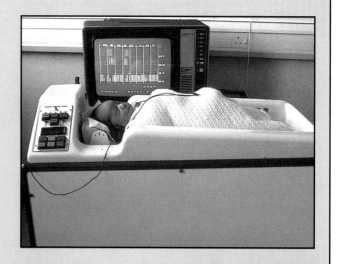

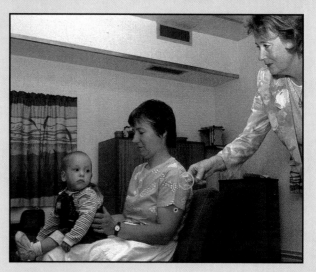

Hearing tests

Older children can take more part in hearing tests. They play special games that make use of their understanding of speech. The tester may give the child a toy and ask the child to "put it in the box" or "give it to Mummy". The levels of sound used in these games are measured with a meter. This helps the tester to discover the most quiet sounds that a child can hear.

At the age of about two years, children can be given a performance test. In this test, the child is asked to put small wooden pieces into a wooden board when the tester says "go". This tests low frequency sounds. A similar test using a hissing sound tests high frequency.

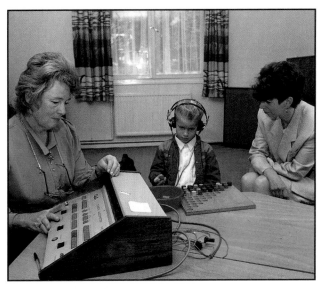

A performance test

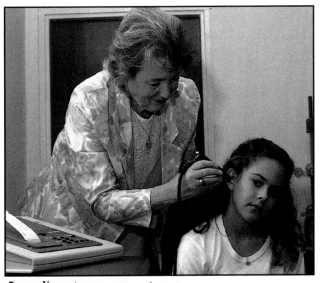

An audiometer measures tones

Pure tone audiometry

From the age of about three years onwards, it is possible to measure hearing more precisely with a test called pure tone audiometry. The person listens through headphones to a series of tones produced by a machine called an audiometer (left). Each tone is a different frequency (pitch). The loudness of the tone is reduced until the person can just hear it.

The results of the test are plotted on a chart called an audiogram. This shows the frequency and loudness of the sounds the person was able to hear. The results for the right ear are plotted as small circles. For the left ear, the results are plotted as crosses.

An Artificial ear

Some babies are born with no ears, and to remedy this condition artificial ears with a special titanium hearing aid implant can be made. First a titanium hearing aid is implanted and integrated into the bone tissue and then the new ear is fitted. The ears look real and allow the patient to feel more confident, wear glasses, swim, play sports and be more easily accepted at school.

In other cases, perhaps after the ear has been badly damaged in an accident, plastic surgery may help. The surgeon uses skin from other parts of the body to reconstruct a replacement outer ear, which allows the hearing system to work as normally as possible.

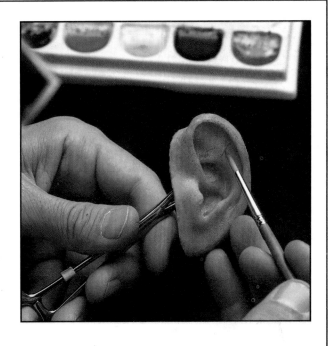

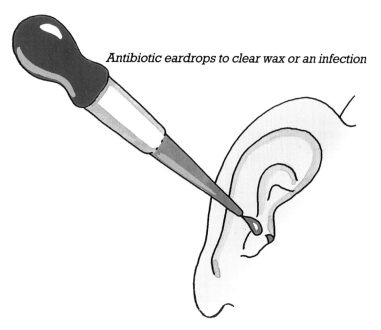

Antibiotic eardrops to clear wax or an infection

Outer ear treatments

If there is too much wax in the ear canal and the wax has become hardened, olive oil drops can be used to soften or dissolve it. The wax will then be able to move out of the ear naturally. It is best to ask a doctor about other kinds of eardrops because they may cause allergic reactions in some people. If the wax continues to be a problem, a doctor can remove it by using a syringe to wash it out. But if syringeing is carried out too often, it seems to reduce the natural process of wax movement. So, after a time, syringeing has to be carried out more and more frequently.

It is not easy to treat an infection in the ear canal, and it is important to treat it before it becomes too serious. An ear infection is more likely to clear up quickly if you consult a doctor as soon as possible. The other important point is to keep the ear dry at all times and avoid scratching the ear. Once the ear is dry, antibiotic eardrops can be used to try and kill off the infection. As with drops that are used to clear wax, some people may be allergic to antibiotic drops.

If a person is born with no ears or only rudimentary ears, or no ear canal, surgeons may be able to operate and try to correct the defect. Operations to create an ear canal are difficult and do not usually restore hearing to a useful level. But the surgeon may be able to make an ear canal that is large enough to take a hearing aid, making it a worthwhile operation.

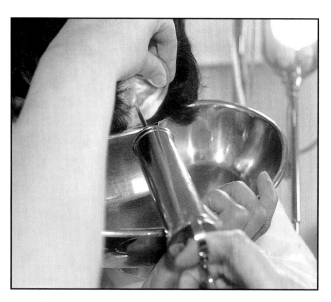

A doctor washing an ear canal with a syringe

Sealing holes in the eardrum

Occasionally, holes in the eardrum do not heal up (right). If this happens, an operation can remedy the problem. A small piece of muscle is joined over the hole, and this grows onto the eardrum to seal it.

If the perforation is too large for this kind of surgery, a whole eardrum can be transplanted. Artificial eardrums may also be used.

Popping in the ears when we descend rapidly in a lift is caused by small movements of the eardrum through changes of pressure in the middle ear. This kind of pressure change is not dangerous and will not normally cause damage to the eardrum.

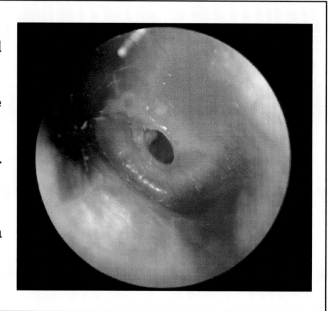

Mastoid surgery

If infections in the middle ear are not cleared up with antibiotics, the infection can spread to the ear bones. Over a long period of time, the infection may even spread to the mastoid bone behind the ear. Once this happens, the bone or part of the bone has to be removed. The middle ear bones may also have to be removed, so this operation does not usually improve hearing. If a cavity is left in the mastoid bone, wax and other debris may collect so the cavity has to be cleaned out from time to time. Mastoid operations are less common nowadays.

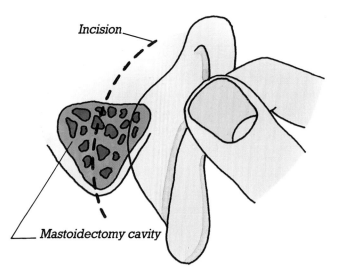

Incision

Mastoidectomy cavity

Grommets

If there is a build-up of fluid in the middle ear, a tiny slit in the eardrum can be made and the infected fluid "sucked out". Sometimes, after the operation a small plastic tube called a grommet, or ventilation tube, is pushed through the slit. This stays in place for up to a year, and allows any more excess fluid to drain away. The grommet eventually falls out of the eardrum and comes out of the ear on its own. The slit in the eardrum usually heals naturally.

Grommets are often inserted when young children suffer with a series of ear infections and the grommet falls out as the ear canal grows and develops naturally as part of the child's development.

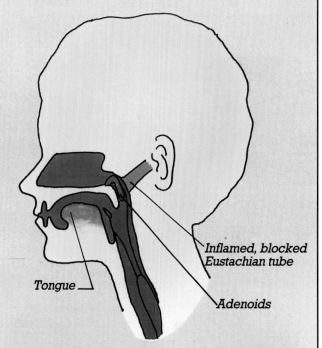

Inflamed, blocked Eustachian tube

Tongue

Adenoids

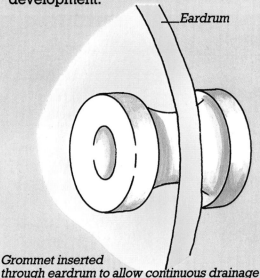

Eardrum

Grommet inserted through eardrum to allow continuous drainage

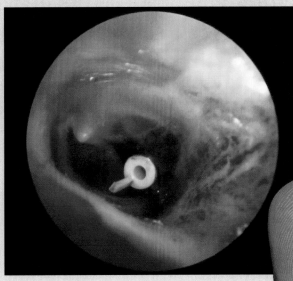

Surgery for ear bone problems

In the recent past there was little doctors could do to help people with problems in the inner part of their ear. But with modern surgical techniques this situation has drastically changed. The disease in which a bony growth stops the middle ear bones from vibrating freely, called otosclerosis, affects many people. The symptoms include a slow onset of deafness, sometimes accompanied by tinnitus. In the first stages of the disease a hearing aid can help the person to hear. But as time goes on, the disease progresses and a hearing aid is no longer useful. For this reason, and because people often suffer from this condition at an early age, surgery is usually carried out.

The original operation to remedy the problem was called a fenestration operation – *fenestra* is Latin for window. A large hole is made in the mastoid bone behind the ear. Sound waves can then bypass the middle ear by travelling through the hole directly to the cochlea in the inner ear. This operation was very successful but has now been replaced by a more successful operation called a stapedectomy (see below).

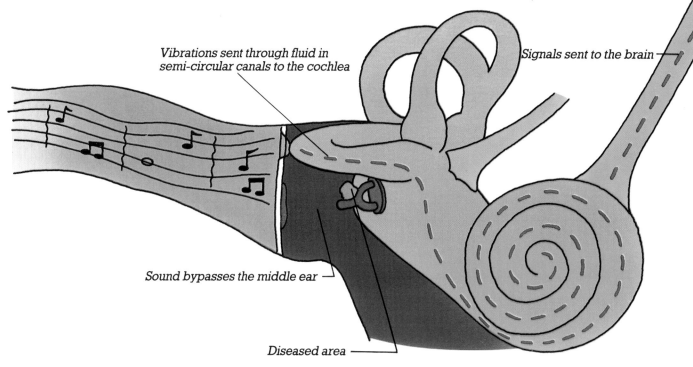

Vibrations sent through fluid in semi-circular canals to the cochlea

Signals sent to the brain

Sound bypasses the middle ear

Diseased area

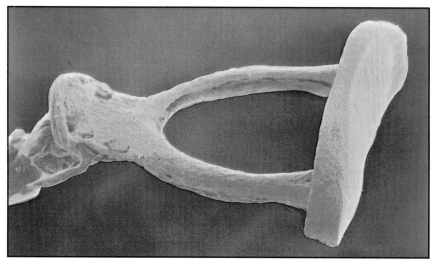

Electron micrograph of a stirrup bone

Stapedectomy

A stapedectomy operation is carried out to remove the stapes (stirrup) bone in the middle ear and replace it with a metal or plastic one. If the operation is not carried out when the ear is affected by otosclerosis, bony growth eventually stops the stapes from vibrating against the oval window. As a result, vibrations do not reach the cochlea in the inner ear.

Cochlear implants

Cochlear implants are minute hearing aids, which are powered by batteries, worn in a speech synthesizer box. During surgery, a tiny electrode is placed on to or inside the cochlea in the inner ear. The electrode is designed to carry an electric current which stimulates the nerve endings in the cochlea.

The current for the electrode comes from an electronic box strapped onto a person's body. This processes the sound picked up by a microphone and passes it to two coils. One coil is behind the ear and the other is under the skin close to the ear. The coils trigger a current in the electrode remotely. They are not connected to the electrode to cut down on the risk of infection.

Cochlear implants divert sound waves straight to the cochlea and can help people who are profoundly deaf. But they can only help a person to recognize sounds, and so are not a cure for deafness.

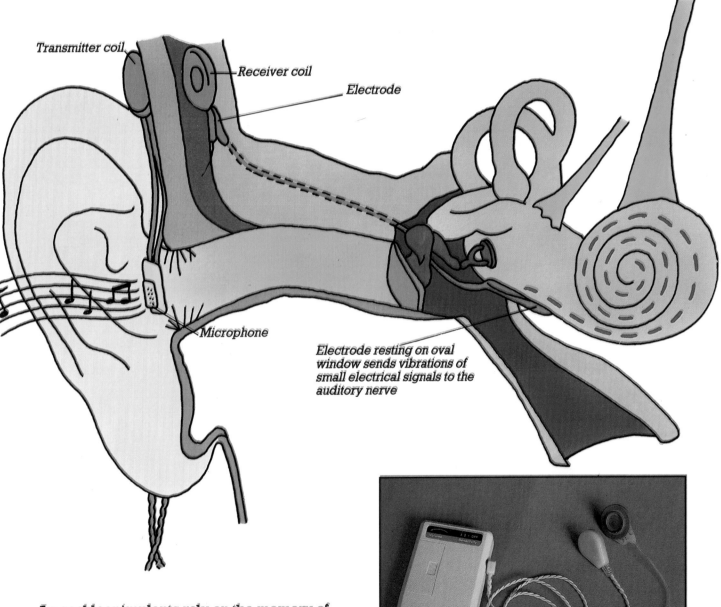

Transmitter coil

Receiver coil

Electrode

Microphone

Electrode resting on oval window sends vibrations of small electrical signals to the auditory nerve

As cochlear implants rely on the memory of sound, there have been very few of these operations performed on children. World-wide, about 3,000 people have received cochlear implants. The diagnosis of deafness is not accurate enough in very young children to justify using cochlear implants.

Sound processor – small box worn on the body

Hearing aids

A hearing aid is designed to pick up sounds and make them louder. It does not make the sounds clearer. Hearing aids that are carried on the body usually make sounds louder than those that are worn behind the ear.

One of the problems with hearing aids is that the batteries need to be replaced frequently, sometimes as often as three times a week. The battery for early hearing aids used to be very large and cumbersome. Fortunately, modern hearing aids have much smaller batteries. Some fit snugly behind the ear in a miniaturized unit and are only about the size of a shirt button. The earmould part of the aid fits inside the ear and feeds sound from the hearing aid down the ear canal to the eardrum. Earmoulds are made from an impression taken of the ear with a soft rubbery substance.

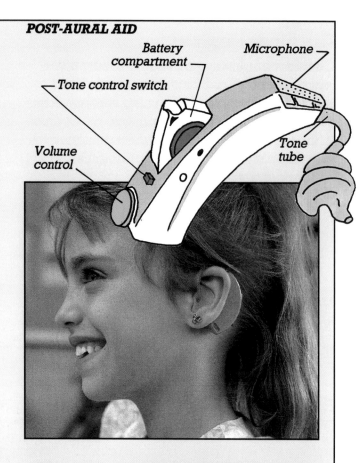

POST-AURAL AID

Battery compartment

Microphone

Tone control switch

Volume control

Tone tube

Loop systems

Loop systems are used in public places, such as theatres (their logo is shown here). They can even be built into a telephone earpiece. A wire loop is connected to the source of a sound, such as a television set.

The wire gives out a magnetic field. This can be picked up by a hearing aid, which converts the magnetic field back into sound. The loop system cuts out background noises and echoes.

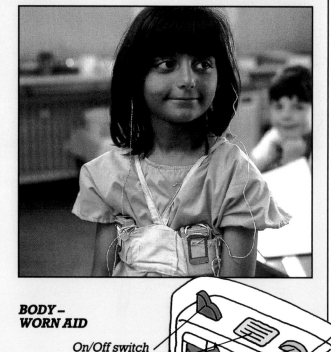

BODY – WORN AID

On/Off switch

Microphone

Volume control

Battery

Amplifier

Receiver

Lead

Radio aids in the classroom

There are often many background noises in a classroom, and this can make it hard for the child to hear what the teacher is saying with an ordinary hearing aid. Sound waves become weaker as they travel through air. Radio aids overcome this problem by using radio waves, which do not lose as much strength as sound waves do when they travel through air. Radio aids are very expensive though, and need to have their batteries charged every night.

Radio aids send sounds directly from one person to another. They are made up of two parts. The teacher wears a radio transmitter linked to a microphone. Radio waves from the transmitter are picked up by a radio receiver, which the child wears. The receiver may also work as a hearing aid and pass louder sounds to the child's ears. Or the receiver may pass the signals on to the child's ordinary hearing aid. In a school, each class may need its own separate frequency or wavelength to tune into, so that a child in one class does not pick up signals from another class.

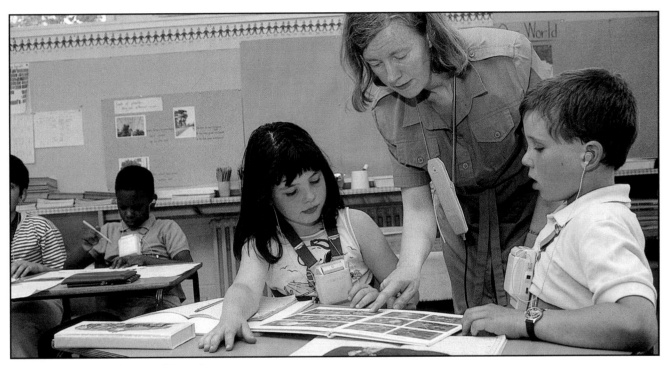

Radiophonic aid being used in a classroom

Tinnitus masker

Small machines that look like hearing aids may help people who suffer from tinnitus (right). These machines are called maskers because they make a gentle, rushing sound that "masks" or covers up the uncomfortable buzzing or ringing noises. The masker is most useful if it makes noises at the same loudness and frequency as the noises in the person's ears or head. It is often very difficult to pin down which are the problem frequencies for a particular person. This is because the noises are something that only the person can hear. Tinnitus maskers basically boost sounds from outside the head which makes the sufferer less aware of the tinnitus. But some people simply have to learn to live with tinnitus.

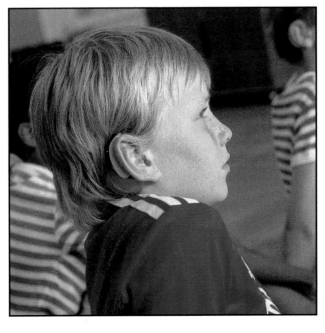

19

LIVING WITH DEAFNESS

If a person finds it hard or even impossible to hear, it is more difficult to cope with everyday life, education, work and leisure activities. The kinds of difficulties depend on the type and amount of deafness. For example, some people cannot hear high frequency sounds, and so cannot hear consonants such as "s", "t", "sh" and "th" in speech. People born with a hearing loss find it very difficult to learn how to speak. It is especially important that they are encouraged to use a variety of methods of communication, including sign language and lipreading and to use hearing aids. If people with a hearing loss are given help and encouragement from a very early age there is no reason why they should not do well at school. Over 80 per cent of children with a hearing impairment do not go to special schools. With care and understanding, from parents and teachers and other social relationships, children that are hard of hearing can achieve a high standard of education.

Everyday living

Many everyday events, such as answering the door bell or getting up on time, cause problems for people with a hearing loss. Some electronic devices may make life easier. These include adaptors that make lights flash or special pads that vibrate when bells ring. Some alarm clocks have a pad that fits under the mattress or pillow and vibrates to wake you up. A telephone can have an amplifier or a loop system (see page 18) fitted. The loop system can be linked to a hearing aid. Another device that helps people that are hard of hearing is a viewdata adaptor. Connected to a telephone line it allows a person to see the information from a telephone call written on a television screen. In the United Kingdom there is a telephone exchange for the deaf where an operator types what the person is saying. The words appear on a screen in the deaf person's home or office. It is perfectly possible for deaf people to lead a normal and useful life. Some authorities even allow partially deaf people to drive – provided warning sounds are converted into visual signals.

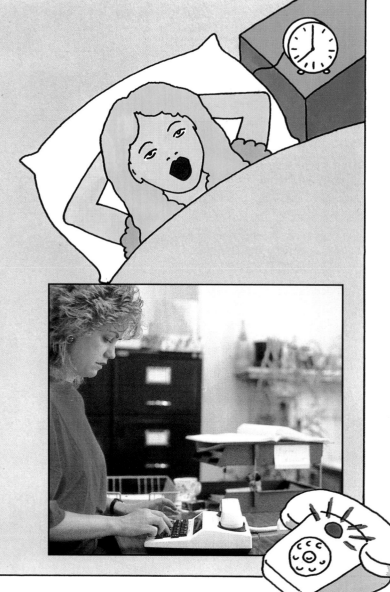

Visual aids

Television has many advantages for people with hearing problems because it can communicate visually. But listening is also important with television. This is often a major problem for a person with a hearing loss. Turning up the volume is not usually the answer because this may irritate other members of the family or neighbours. In some countries, a small percentage of programmes have subtitles or captions and sign language so that deaf people will find the information easier to follow and understand. If subtitles were available on more television programmes, it would make it much easier for deaf people to enjoy watching television.

Some television channels show electronic "magazines" of information with words and diagrams on all sorts of topics, such as news, travel, finance and sport. There may be special "magazines" for people with a hearing loss. These may include a summary of a play or drama series which will be appearing on television in the near future or news (above right). This sort of preparation helps deaf people to follow the action more easily. You need a special type of television to receive these magazine programmes.

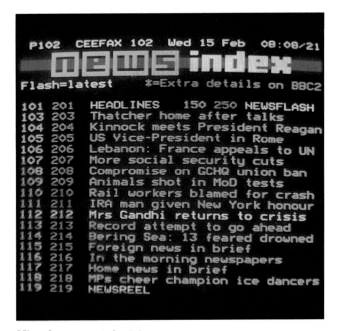

Visual news on television

Many televisions have a socket that takes headphones, a special microphone or an infra-red listening device. You can also have a loop system (see page 18) fitted in the home so you can listen to the television through a hearing aid. With a loop system, you can hear the television as if the sound were coming straight from the loudspeaker. But you will not hear background noise, such as other people talking in the room.

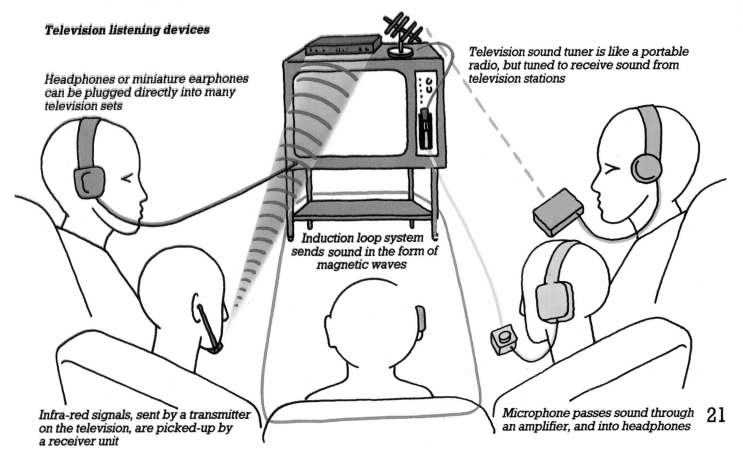

Television listening devices

Headphones or miniature earphones can be plugged directly into many television sets

Television sound tuner is like a portable radio, but tuned to receive sound from television stations

Induction loop system sends sound in the form of magnetic waves

Infra-red signals, sent by a transmitter on the television, are picked-up by a receiver unit

Microphone passes sound through an amplifier, and into headphones

21

Fingerspelling and sign language

Fingerspelling is a language that uses hand and finger shapes to represent the letters of the alphabet. This is called a manual alphabet. Throughout the world, there are many types of manual alphabet. Many, such as the American version, use one hand. This leaves the other hand free for other tasks. Other manual alphabets, such as the British one, use two hands.

With practice, you can learn fingerspelling very quickly. Fingerspelling can be used as a way of communicating by touch with people who are both deaf and blind. Sign language is a different sort of language that uses hand shapes and hand movements as well as eye movements, facial expressions and body positions to stand for whole words or ideas.

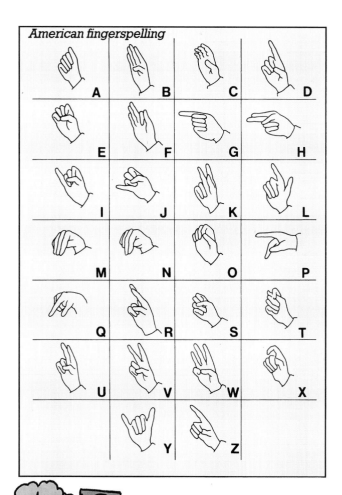

American fingerspelling

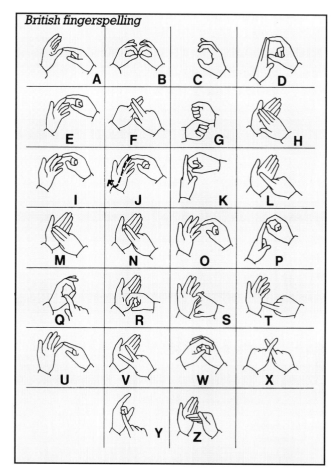

British fingerspelling

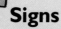

Signs

Signs for words or ideas are made with the hands but meaning is also given by the expression of the face and position of the body. It takes a long time to learn how to sign well. There are different sign languages in different countries.

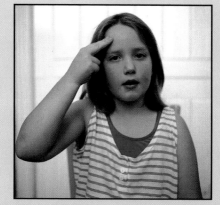

Name

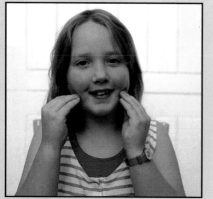

Thankyou

Lipreading or speech reading

A person with a hearing loss may be able to work out the sounds a person is making by "reading" the shape of the lips. This is called lipreading or speech reading. The technique can be of some use if the speaker forms the words clearly. But even the best lipreader probably reads only 50 per cent of the words spoken. The rest is just guesswork. Many sounds in the English language are invisible on the lips. For example, the difference between the words "goal" and "coal" depend only on sounds made in the throat. Other sounds, such as "p", "b" and "m", "d" and "n" and "s" and "z" can be easily confused. If you do not know much about the subject of a conversation, lipreading is even more difficult. For a person who has been born deaf, lipreading is much more difficult than for a person that used to be able to hear. This is because a deaf person has to imagine sounds that have never been heard.

Deafness or even a slight hearing impairment can lead to a loss of confidence and a feeling of being shut out from everyday living. As a result, deafness can be a considerable social barrier as no one willingly stays in a situation in which he or she feels ill at ease.

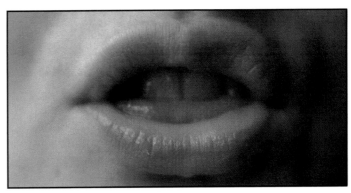
Lips making a "th" sound

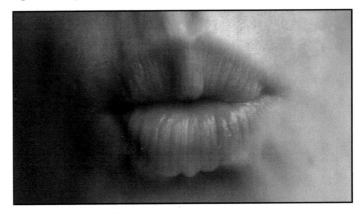
Lips making an "o" sound

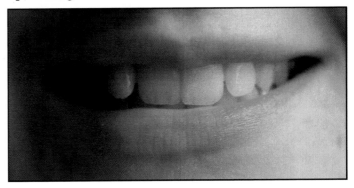
Lips making an "e" sound

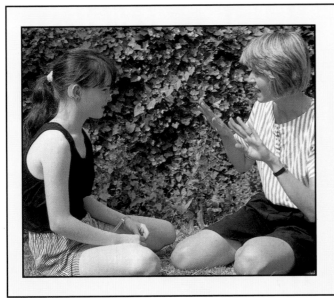

Conversation

To help a deaf person to lipread, you should make sure that he or she can see your face clearly all the time. Do not stand in shadow or with your back to a bright light. You should talk naturally but not too slowly and speak as clearly as possible. It is not helpful to shout because this distorts the mouth patterns and makes lipreading more difficult. While you are talking, do not eat or smoke and avoid putting your hand over your mouth. Try to appreciate how difficult lipreading is and be prepared to repeat words.

Learning to speak

Like all children, deaf children are born with the ability to learn and develop language. But deaf children find it difficult to learn speech because they have to imitate sounds they can see rather than sounds they can hear. And it is very difficult to control the sounds you make if you cannot hear the sound of your own voice.

A machine that lights up to show the loudness of speech helps deaf people to "see" the sounds they make and learn how to control them. Feeling the throat while speaking can also be helpful. The vibrations made by sounds give clues to how loud they are and when they are changing which help a child learn to speak.

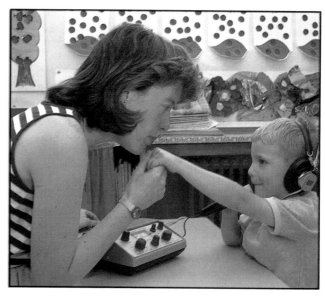

Helping a deaf child become aware of sounds

Feeling the vibrations

If you hold a balloon near your mouth as you speak, you will feel the balloon vibrating. This happens because the balloon picks up the sound waves your voice makes. A balloon can be used to help a deaf child learn how to control the voice. The teacher speaks into the balloon and the deaf child feels the vibrations. The child then tries to make a sound which causes the same vibration.

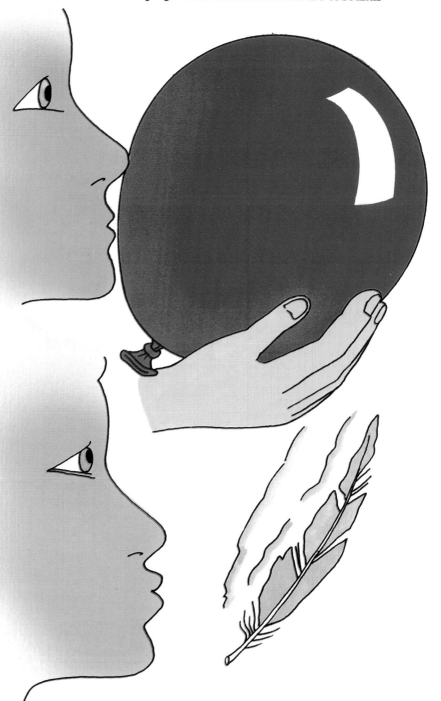

Breath control

The noises we make when speaking are made by passing air over the vocal cords. The noises also depend on how we control the air with our lips and tongue. So to speak clearly it is very important to be able to control your breathing. Deaf people can practise a number of different exercises, such as blowing a feather, to try and improve their breathing and have control over it.

24

Music

Children with a hearing loss have a range of interests and abilities. Depending on the level of their hearing loss, there is no reason why they should not enjoy music. Deaf people can feel sound vibrations and rhythms through musical instruments. Many learn to play musical instruments. Some partially deaf children are able to hear more high pitched notes well. As the ear is also the organ of balance, some kinds of deafness may affect a person's sense of balance and some people, particularly young children, tend to be more accident prone because of this.

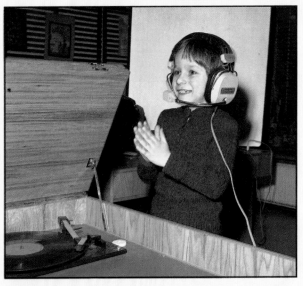

Feeling rhythm through music

Losing the sense of sound

The brain begins to amass a store of sound memories from the moment of birth, and by adulthood people are able to distinguish nearly half a million signals that are meaningful. Should the sound memory centre be accidentally destroyed, a condition called auditory amnesia occurs. Although nerve impulses corresponding to sounds do reach the brain, they no longer have any meaning. This is a difficult condition to treat because it is the brain, rather than the ear itself, that is damaged.

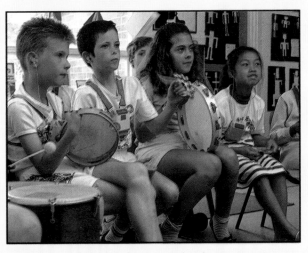

Feeling sound through percussion instruments

Dance

Deaf children can appreciate natural rhythms, even if they are profoundly deaf. So they may enjoy dancing and this can also help them to learn how to co-ordinate their movements. A loop system (see page 21) can help partially deaf children in this activity. It allows hearing aids to be used like a radio receiver. Music can be wired so that it is picked up by the children's hearing aid.

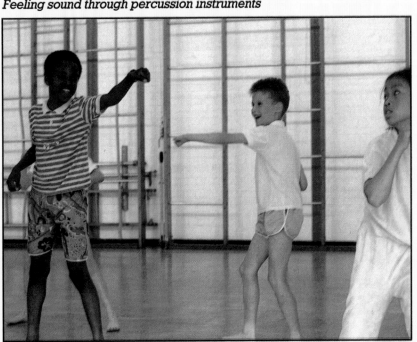

Dance therapy helps co-ordination and balance

DEAFNESS AND SOCIETY

Children with a hearing loss are educated in ordinary schools as far as possible. Generally, the choice regarding the kind of education that a child with a hearing loss has is made according to parental preference – in the same way as any child's education. There are special schools available for children with hearing disabilities. In special schools the education is as wide as in ordinary schools but it is delivered by teachers who have had some training in the use of hearing aids and other equipment, as well as the use of sign language. Alternatively, some special schools maximize on the residual hearing of the pupils and use hearing aids without any signing systems such as sign language.

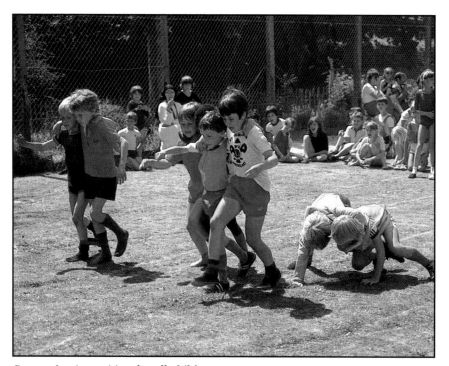

Sports day is exciting for all children

At school

In some special schools for deaf children the teaching methods incorporate all kinds of communication – signing systems and hearing aids. Using "total communication" methods, deaf children are free to choose the best way of expressing their ideas and feelings. Deaf children have to work harder than hearing children in order to keep up with their lessons and so they are under more stress. Teachers should make allowances for this, and we all should be aware of emotional and social difficulties.

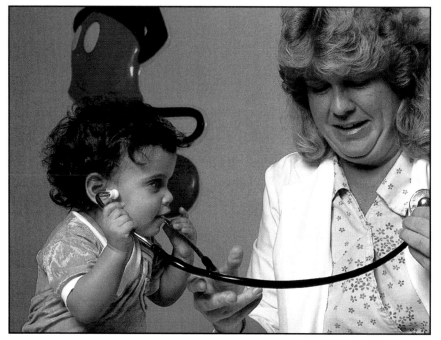

At work

There are many occasions when deaf people find an interpreter useful. These include telephone calls, job interviews, medical or dental examinations and conferences

At home

The early formative years are vital for a child who is born deaf or has hearing problems. The family should try and help the child feel safe and comfortable so he or she is able to relax in a world without sound.

A young child using a stethoscope as an amplifier

LEADING A NORMAL LIFE

Approximately one child in every thousand is born profoundly deaf and mild or partial hearing loss is not unusual. It is important for everyone to understand that deaf children are certainly not dumb but they simply have difficulty in learning to speak. This is because they cannot hear other people's voices or their own – which is why their voices often sound strange. The more aware that people are towards the particular difficulties that deaf people encounter, the easier it is to adjust to the problems. In adults, the deafness caused by a gradual hearing loss in old age simply increases feelings of loneliness and isolation. Although deafness is a handicap, it is possible, particularly with help and care from others, for deaf people to lead a normal life. For young babies who are born with deafness, the world may seem to be a hard and frightening place to understand at first. But if a baby is stimulated during the first few formative years of life, he or she will probably grow up to be as well-adjusted and have the same kind of opportunities as other children who can hear and are not deaf.

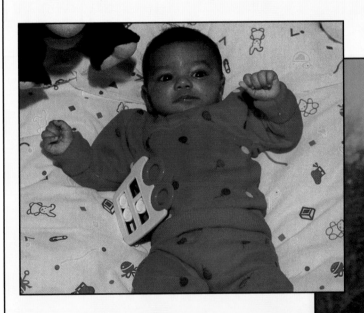

Helping to communicate

When you speak to someone who is using a hearing aid, consider the problems they might have. It is important to cut down outside noise by shutting doors and windows. Face the person, keep your hands from your face and speak directly, because your listener may also be lipreading. It is important to speak slowly and distinctly – do not shout as this overloads the amplifier and distorts sound. Also try to avoid unnecessary background noises such as jangling keys and money.

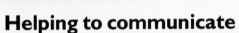

CARING FOR YOUR EARS

Many sounds can damage your hearing, including noisy aircraft, industrial machines and very loud music. If you are exposed to loud noise for a short while, you may feel slightly deaf for a time. But your hearing should slowly return to normal when you are out of the noisy environment. Too much loud noise, however, can lead to a permanent hearing loss.

A person firing a gun or using a chain saw should wear ear muffs to protect the ears. It is also a good idea to protect your ears if you use a noisy electric drill in a small space or for a long time. People in noise-producing occupations such as a road drill operator are at risk if they do not protect their ears from constant noise.

People often do not like to wear ear muffs or ear plugs because it cuts them off from other people and things around them. Some people's ears are more at risk than others, but it is impossible to find this out until damage has already occurred.

Decibels

The loudness of sound is measured in units called decibels, or dB for short. Sixty dB is the loudness of conversation, and 120 dB that of a jet engine. If a person "loses" 25 dB of loudness, he or she may have a hearing difficulty. A loss of 95 dB can make a person almost totally deaf.

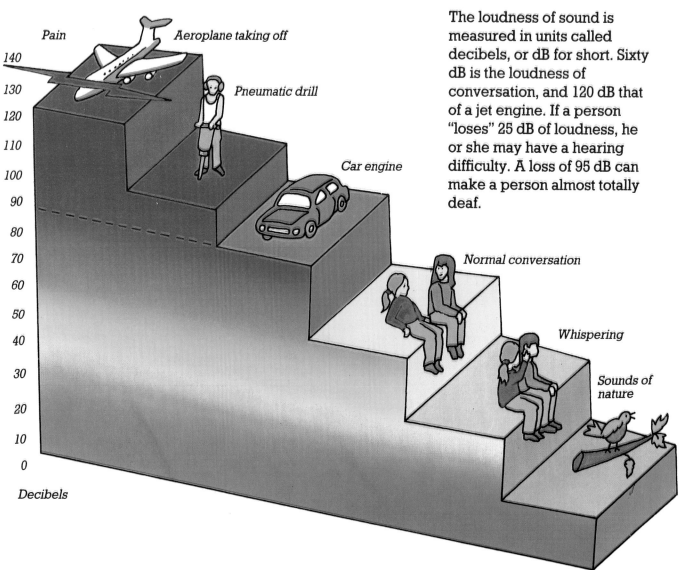

Pain — Aeroplane taking off — Pneumatic drill — Car engine — Normal conversation — Whispering — Sounds of nature

140 130 120 110 100 90 80 70 60 50 40 30 20 10 0

Decibels

Noise at work

Working in very noisy factories and industries impairs many people's hearing. The loud noise damages the sensitive cochlea in the inner ear. It is not just the amount of noise that is important, but also the length of time you are close to it. Laws have been passed to set the level above which a noise becomes dangerous. This is 90 dB in the United Kingdom and 85 dB in the United States. If the noise is above this limit, employers should provide ear plugs or ear muffs. Safety officers check that ear protection is available and is being used in the correct way.

Loud music

Constant bombardment of the ears with loud music at discotheques and pop concerts can also cause loss of hearing. Even the quieter modern bands can produce sound levels that are dangerously high. The noise level in an average discotheque can be as high as 120 dB – the same as from a jet aircraft. The people most likely to suffer are those running the shows because they have to listen to the loud noise night after night. Playing music too loudly on a personal stereo for long periods of time can also damage a person's ears. This kind of problem can easily be avoided.

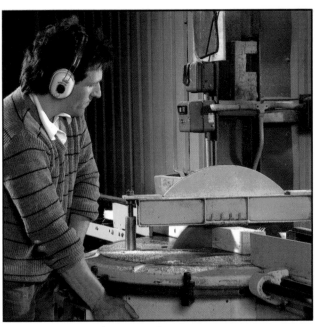

Wear ear protection at work

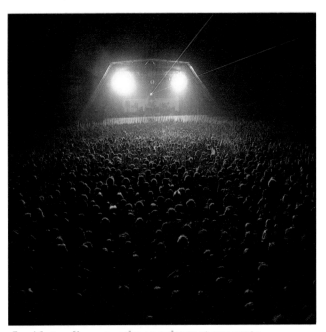

Avoid standing near the speakers at concerts

In the water

If a person has a perforated eardrum or grommets (see page 15) in the eardrum, he or she should try to avoid water in their ears. If the water reaches the middle ear, it could cause infections or damage the ear. Wearing a swimming cap helps to prevent water reaching into the ears, especially if the person keeps the head above water. There is a silicon putty that a person can squeeze into their ear which creates a watertight seal. Used with a swimming cap it provides good protection against ear infections.

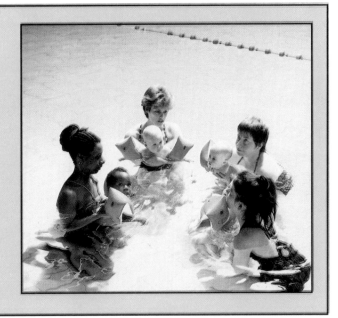

FIRST AID

You should never push or poke anything into your ears to try and clean the ear canal. This can compress the ear wax into a hard lump and stop it moving out of the ear as it should naturally. The job of ear wax is to trap dirt and debris and carry it out of the ear. So if you leave your ears alone, they will clean themselves. There is also a risk that poking things into the ear may damage the eardrum and cause serious hearing problems.

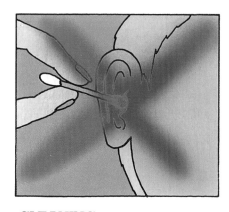

CLEANING
There is usually no need to clean your ears. The hairs and wax in the ear canal will do the job for you.

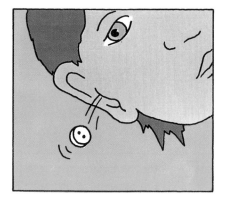

FOREIGN BODIES
If an object does become stuck in the ear canal, tilt the head to let it fall out and go to a doctor for help.

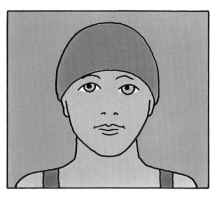

SWIMMING
If you have any ear problems, wear a cap when you go swimming.

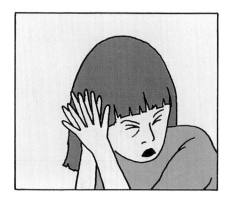

EARACHE
If you have an earache, you should go to a doctor for treatment as soon as possible.

Earaches are a sign that something is wrong with the ear. They can be caused by such things as infections in the middle ear. This can lead to more serious disorders as the infection can spread to other parts of the body. Therefore, the sooner treatment can begin, the safer it is for you and the rest of the family. If you have any problems with your ears, go to a doctor for a check-up as soon as you can.

People to contact

The National Deaf Children's Society,
45 Hereford Road,
London W2 5AH.
Tel: 01-229-9272.
Information on all issues concerning deaf children.

The Royal National Institute for the Deaf (RNID),
105 Gower Street,
London WC1E 6AH.
Tel: 01-387-8033.
Information and help to deaf people and training for profoundly deaf people.

The British Deaf Association,
38 Victoria Place,
Carlisle CA1 1HU.
Tel: Carlisle (0228) 48844.
Information on sign language, interpreting and education.

The British Association of the Hard of Hearing,
7-11 Armstrong Road,
London W3 7JL.
Tel: 01-743-1110.

GLOSSARY

Audiogram A chart showing the amount of hearing loss in decibels.

Auditory nerve The nerve that carries electrical signals (nerve impulses) from the cochlea to the brain.

Cochlea A bony structure in the inner ear which converts the frequency and loudness of sound into electrical signals.

Cochlear implants Tiny hearing aids which are implanted onto or inside the cochlea.

Conductive deafness A hearing impairment which affects the outer or middle ear. It can often be treated.

Decibel A unit used to measure the loudness of sound.

Earmould A piece of plastic, moulded to fit the shape of the ear, which conducts sound from a hearing aid into the ear.

Eustachian tube A tube leading from the middle ear to the throat.

Fingerspelling Using hand and finger shapes to stand for the letters of the alphabet.

Frequency (pitch) Sound vibrations per second, measured in hertz (Hz).

Glue ear A build-up of thick, sticky fluid in the middle ear, due to a blocked Eustachian tube.

Grommet A small plastic tube used to hold open a slit in the eardrum.

Hearing aid A device which makes sounds louder. It may be worn behind the ear (post-aural aid), on spectacles, on the body (body-worn aid) or in the ear.

Lipreading Trying to understand speech by "reading" the shape of the lips. It is sometimes called speech reading.

Loop system A wire loop connected to the source of a sound. It gives out a magnetic field which a hearing aid converts back into sound again.

Myringoplasty An operation to repair a hole in the eardrum.

Nerve deafness This condition is also sometimes referred to as sensori-neural deafness. It is a hearing impairment which affects the inner ear or pathways to the brain. It causes distortion of speech and makes speech hard to understand. It cannot usually be treated medically.

Otosclerosis A condition in which the middle ear bones become covered with a bony growth and cannot vibrate freely.

Oval window The entrance to the inner ear. The interface between the ossicles and fluid-filled cochlea in the inner ear.

Pure tone audiometry A way of testing how well a person can hear a range of tones of one frequency only.

Radio aid A device which sends radio waves from one person to another. A radio receiver or a hearing aid converts the radio waves into sound waves and makes them louder.

Sign language A system of signs made with the hands. The signs stand for words or ideas.

Total communication A way of teaching that uses all forms of communication, including sign language, fingerspelling, speech reading, lipreading, drawing and writing.

INDEX

Photographic Credits:
Cover and page 29b: Anthea Sieveking/Network; pages 5, 22 and 23: Roger Vlitos; pages 6, 10, 11 all, 16, 21, 29t and 29m: Science Photo Library; page 7: Magnum Photos; pages 8, 14 and 15 both: National Medical Slide Bank; pages 10 and 14: Biophoto Associates; pages 12 both, 13 all, 17, 18 all, 19 both, 20, 23, 24 and 25m and 25b: Janine Weidel; page 25t: Zefa; page 26: J. Allan Cash Library; pages 26 and 27t: Robert Harding; pages 27m and 27b: Images/Biophot Associates.